How to Control
Asthma and Allergy

Dr RAJEEV SHARMA

NEW DAWN PRESS, INC.
USA• UK• INDIA

NEW DAWN PRESS GROUP

Published by New Dawn Press Group

New Dawn Press, Inc., 244 South Randall Rd # 90, Elgin, IL 60123
e-mail: sales@newdawnpress.com

New Dawn Press, 2 Tintern Close, Slough, Berkshire, SL1-2TB, UK
e-mail: salesuk@newdawnpress.org

New Dawn Press (An Imprint of Sterling Publishers (P) Ltd)
A-59, Okhla Industrial Area, Phase-II, New Delhi-110020, India
e-mail: info@sterlingpublishers.com
www.sterlingpublishers.com

How to Control Asthma and Allergy
© 2006, Sterling Publishers (P) Ltd
ISBN 1 84557 534 2

PRINTED IN INDIA

Contents

	Publisher's Note	5
1.	The Lungs .	6
2.	Causes and Types of Asthma	12
3.	Asthma in Children	16
4.	Treatment by Alternative Systems	21
5.	Treatment by Naturopathy and Yogic Exercise	27
6.	Treatment by Allopathy	41
7.	Diet	49
8.	Frequently Asked Questions	55
9.	Some Objective Questions	62
10.	Enlarged Tonsils and Asthma	66
11.	Perennial Sneezing or Perennial Allergic Rhinitis	69
12.	Seasonal Sneezing or Hay Fever	80
13.	Allergy to Drugs	84

Contents

Publisher's Note

Asthma and Allergy is an easy-to-read reference book. It is intended as a home advisor but is not a substitute for a doctor.

The opinions are those of the author, and the publisher holds no responsibility.

This particular book is an authentic work of Dr Rajeev Sharma author of more than 125 books of general interest, related to the field of medicine.

The Lungs

In order to understand asthma, we first need to understand a little about the normal structure and function of the lungs.

The most important function of the lungs is taking in of oxygen from the air into the blood stream and getting rid of the waste carbon dioxide. In order to do this, air has to be brought very close to the blood and this happens in tiny air sacs called alveoli. These alveoli are the end of an extensive branching structure which starts with trachea, the main airway into the lung.

Blood from the veins (from all over the body) drains into the right side of the heart and is then pumped through the lungs by way of the tiny vessels in the walls of the alveoli. There, it picks up oxygen (oxygenation of blood) and gets rid of carbon dioxide before returning to the left side of the heart. Oxygenated blood from the left side of the heart is pumped out to all the tissues in the body through the arteries.

The airways

Various objects, including liquids and food particles, can enter the lungs via trachea. The large airways such as the trachea have a stiff wall, which contains cartilage, the same substance as that supports our nose and ears. These are present in the form of a ring. This is present only in the anterior and is absent in the posterior. This makes these large airways less likely to narrow in asthma. In children, of course, all the airways are smaller. All the airways are lined by an epithelium, which is like a thin skin, and on the top of this skin are tiny hairs called cilia which are constantly in motion shifting up the lung secretions from the outer portions of the lungs to the large airways. Underneath the epithelia layer, there is a loose mass of tissue called connective tissue in which there are two important structures, the bronchial glands and the smooth muscle.

The bronchial glands

These have little tubes opening on to the inner surface of the airway. Through these, they pour secretions of mucus into the airway where again it is wafted up in the larger airways and then coughed up as abnormally sticky sputum. This adds to the narrowing of the airways and may play a crucial role in asthma patients. These thick and tenacious mucus plugs that block most of the airways, constitute the most remarkable feature in the lungs of patients who die of asthma.

Smooth muscle

The bronchi has smooth muscles wrapped around it like stripes on a candy stick. The state of tension of these muscles is an important factor in determining the diameter of the bronchus; contraction of bronchial muscles narrows the bronchus, while relaxation widens it.

Inspiration and expiration

Breathing in is also known as inspiration (inhalation) and breathing out is called expiration (exhalation). Under normal circumstances, little work is required for the breathing process. However, there are two things that make this work much harder and difficult:

- stiffness of the lungs
- narrowing of the airways

Bronchial reactivity

Increased bronchial reactivity in asthma is related to airway inflammation in which many cells participate. These include mast cells. Previously, it was believed that mast cells are crucial in the pathogenesis of bronchial asthma. However, it has been shown recently that other cells also participate. These are eosinophils, lymphocytes, macrophages, neutrophils and platelets, etc. These cells release various mediators which are responsible for symptoms of bronchial asthma. One such mediator released from mast cells is histamine, which produces immediate symptoms (acute bronchospasm or wheezing) of bronchial asthma.

Mediators released from other cells result in bronchial hyper-responsiveness, as a result of which, asthmatic airways exhibit an exaggerated response to agents such as pollen, often manifesting as increased non-specific reactivity for days or even weeks. Upper respiratory tract viral infection may lead to similar changes and may increase reactivity in non-asthmatic subjects.

Lungs and airways in asthma

When the air passage is narrow, as in asthma, the lung it seems tries to keep the airway lumen as wide as possible by keeping more air in the lungs, this is called over inflammation or hyper-inflation. It means that there is less room for air with each breath and breathing in becomes difficult. Breathing out is also limited by the narrow airways. Asthmatics, during an acute attack, usually find it most comfortable to sit up so that their main muscle of respiration (the diaphragm) works best and they may even use extra muscles in the neck to help their breathing.

Typical changes which involve the airways in asthmatics include: inflammation, bronchospasm and mucus production.

Inflammation

Researchers have paid much attention to contraction of the smooth muscle (broncho-constriction) in asthma. In fact, it was considered to be the crucial feature of bronchial asthma and all treatment modalities in the past were directed at reversing this broncho-constriction.

Currently, infiltrating of the airway wall by various inflammatory cells is considered the key abnormality in the pathogenesis of bronchial asthma. Bronchoconstriction is certainly important; but so is the swelling of the airway wall by various inflammatory cells. It is composed of fluid and cells which release various substances that attract other cells. This causes more swelling and leads to contraction of the muscle. Research work has revealed that this inflammation persists to some degree in the walls of airways of asthmatics even when the disease has not given any trouble for 6 to 12 months. These cells lie quietly in the airway wall, waiting for the right stimulus to activate them again and spark off an attack of asthma. Corticosteroid medications are used to reduce this inflammation. Inhaled steroids may prevent it.

Inflammatory cells

Many kinds of inflammatory cells in the wall of the airway are important in asthma. Those which have been best studied are the mast cells. These little packages contain performed mediators which are released if these cells are triggered, for instance, by a pollen grain. Other cells include eosinophils, lymphocytes, platelets, neutrophils and so on.

Bronchospasm

Another characteristic of asthma is increased sensitivity of the airways. This leads to bronchospasm, due to spasm of the smooth muscle around the airways. It causes further narrowing of the airways. Bronchodilator drugs are very effective in reversing this muscle spasm.

Mucus production

In some asthmatics, the mucous glands in the airways produce excessive, thick mucus which further narrows the airways. Cortiocosteroids decrease swelling, thereby lessening mucus production. Drinking adequate fluids and deep coasting can also help to remove the mucus. Expectorants (medications which increase sputum production), and mycologist (medications which loosen the secretion) may also be beneficial.

Causes and Types of Asthma

It is a disease of lungs accompanied by cough and difficult breathing. There is violent oppression of breathing due to spasm and swelling of air passage.

General causes

According to Ayurveda, *Svasa Roga* (asthma) is caused by the violation of *Vata* and *Kapha doshas*. So, causes of *Vata* and *Kapha* are also the causes of asthma.

1. Causes of vitiation of *Vata*: Cold water, excessive exercise, fasting, weakness, intake of dry and contaminated food, suppression of natural urges, inhalation of dust smoke, excessive intercourse, etc.

2. Causes of vitiation of *Kapha*: Intake of excessive and heavy, oily food, use of curd, meat of aquatic animals specially sea food and sesame oil.

3. Other diseases causing asthma: Anaemia, diarrhoea, vomiting, rhinitis, tuberculosis, scurvy, cholera and bronchitis are some of the diseases for which asthma is considered a symptom. In heart diseases,

ascites, gout, cirrhosis of liver and kidney disorders, asthma is taken as a secondary symptom.

4. Certain allergies caused by pollen, food items, fungi, animals might lead to asthma.

Some other precipitatory factors may be sudden, coincidental or situation-based or some may be even specific to a person only in a given situation but disappear as soon as the agonising situation becomes non-existent.

Other causes of asthma

Following factors may also cause asthma, apart from the ones already mentioned:

- Occupation
- Heredity
- Climate
- Emotional Status
- Infection

Types of asthma

Intrinsic asthma

This type of asthma develops due to some pre-existing disease, like some residue of infection or existing disease like bronchitis. Such type of patients do not benefit from or respond to anti-allergic treatment and thus, not easy to manage and control. This variety occurs mostly in advanced age.

Extrinsic asthma

Extrinsic asthma usually and commonly occurs in earlier part of one's life and generally responds to anti-allergic medication and treatment. The underlying cause can be attributed to exposure to allergic agents like certain fungi, house-dust, etc. The patient has an inherited tendency when he gets exposed to the said allergens. Recurring bouts of rhinites (sneezing) and eczema could also be the pre-disposing and precipitory cause to trigger an attack of asthma.

Exercise induced asthma

This type of asthma commonly occurs in those who do physical exercises in the cold weather. But then, all persons may be either partially or not at all affected and some may be having serious manifestations.

Problems relating to asthma can be easily managed in young adults, but extremely difficult to manage in case of elderly and small children.

Important symptoms of asthma

Cough, rattling during inspiration, spasm and heaviness in the chest and respiratory problem.

Asthmatic patients

Following situations and type of persons could be termed as potential patients of asthma:
- Those who generally suffer from throat infection and there is recurrence of symptoms
- Those having a family history of asthma

- Who often suffer from bouts of sneezing, especially at the change of season
- Persons experiencing coughing at the change of season
- Those living in polluted environments and whose houses are dark, damp and filthy, where the standard of personal hygiene is poor and where sunrays cannot enter
- Persons working in cloth mills, chemical factories, flour mills, paint and varnish factories, coal miners, labourers who work in stone quarries
- Who easily get breathless even after a light exercise
- Who are sensitive to cold winds

Asthma in Children

Asthma manifests itself differently in children, adults and elderly people. In children, it is usually manifested as cough and wheeze.

Asthma often starts in childhood, but its presentation then is different from what is observed in adulthood. In children, generally, asthma is present as recurrent attacks of cough and wheezing only. In some attacks, it is accompanied by fever and breathlessness also. Breathlessness in asthmatic children, usually, does not come in the form of paroxysmal attack.

This picture of asthma has to be recognised clearly, otherwise the time lost in making a correct diagnosis leads to the danger of developing chest deformities.

Premonitory symptoms
Children who have allergic symptoms are more liable to get asthma. These symptoms are
- unusual and persistent colic;
- need for frequent changes of feeding formulas;
- unexplained diarrhoea or constipation;
- extreme likes and dislikes for certain foods;

16

- excessive vomiting;
- unexplained skin rashes;
- discharge of pus from the ears (otitis media);
- if one or both the parents have some allergic disorder, there is a likelihood that some of their children may also have it, perhaps, in the form of asthma.

Treatment

Usual bronchodilator drugs, as given in adults, are useful in children as well, except, that they have to be given in reduced dosages, according to the age and weight of the child. For children, these drugs come in the form of liquids or syrups, and so, are easily accepted. If necessary, a liquid preparation of salbutamol is usually adequate in mild cases.

Corticosteroids are rarely required if all other measures are taken adequately. But in case an attack of asthma does not subside in spite of other measures being taken, there is a need for giving cortisone for a few days in order to bring the child out of the attack; cortisone can then be tapered off in a few days time.

It is not advisable to give antibiotics to children unless there is clear evidence of infection. Unnecessary administration of antibiotics like tetracycline are liable to colour teeth permanently. Even though milk teeth fall out, the permanent ones which are already being formed can become discoloured; this has particularly a damaging effect. Penicillin is more liable to cause reactions in allergic children than in others. Hence antibiotics in asthmatic children should only be given when there is clear evidence of a bacterial infection.

Finding out what the child is allergic to and subsequent hypo-sensitisation, if the allergen cannot be eliminated from the diet, is a possible solution. However, it is difficult to get cooperation from children.

Does wheezing always mean asthma?

A case of wheezing and breathlessness may or may not be a case of bronchial asthma. There are other diseases in which wheezing and breathlessness are main or subsidiary symptoms. These conditions need to be recognised properly.

It is necessary to differentiate asthma from acute bronchiolitis, the presence of a foreign body in the bronchial tree, pressure on the main bronchi from a tuberculous gland, an enlarged thymus pressing upon the trachea, bronchiectasis, cystic fibrosis of the pancreas in which lung involvement is predominant, and congenital disease of the heart.

When a foreign body in the respiratory tract causes wheezing and difficulty in breathing, the onset is sudden and there is usually an incidence of having inhaled a foreign material earlier also.

Without a proper and adequate investigation, a wheeze should not be invariably considered as asthma.

Help your Child fight asthma

- Always encourage them to take part in normal day-to-day activities.

- To boost their self-confidence, encourage them to do the things they enjoy most.
- Encourage your child to be as independent as possible.
- As your child grows older, teach him/her about asthma.
- Teach them to be responsible about taking medicines regularly.
- They should know whom to call in case of an emergency.
- Make sure you inform the school authorities about your child's asthma.

Frequently Asked Questions

Will my child outgrow asthma?

Some children outgrow their asthma as they approach their teens, or even earlier. In others, attacks could persist, or stop for a few years and then reappear.

Will my other children also get asthma?

Asthma is not contagious. Someone who has it cannot pass it on to others. Though the tendency to have asthma runs in families, this does not mean that if one of your children has asthma, the others will necessarily get it.

Can my child exercise?

It is important for children with asthma to take part in exercise programmes that increase their physical tolerance without aggravating asthma. If it interferes with their breathing, inform your doctor. He can prescribe appropriate medicines. Swimming and yoga are excellent for children with asthma. Breathing exercises may also be helpful.

Does emotional stress play a part in my child's asthma attack?

Excitement, anger and frustration can aggravate an attack in an asthmatic child. Family problems may also make his condition worse. A positive and confident attitude in parents can go a long way in helping a child with asthma.

Should my child go on a special diet?

Very little is known about the influence of diet on asthma. If you notice that a certain type of food makes your child's asthma worse, avoid it completely. In infants, breastfeeding helps to build up immunity to diseases.

What should I do when my child starts going to school?

It is important not to hide your child's asthma from the teacher. Discuss the symptoms and treatment with the teacher. Make sure your child carries the necessary medicine to school.

Is it safe for my child to go on school trips?

Yes, as long as the asthma is under control. Your child must carry the prescribed medicine, including medicine for a severe attack. It is also very important to remind the accompanying teacher about your child's asthma.

Treatment by Alternative Systems

Homeopathic treatments
The following are some of the medicines in the case of specified symptoms.

Acute state

Bry 30
Inflammation of the wind pipe and mucous membrane, hawking up cough with much less phlegm, blocked nose, watery eyes, digestive problems and burning sensation can be cured by this.

Nux Vom-3
Blocking of one nostril at night.

Ars ALB 30
This is useful in case of frequent sneezing, watering from eyes, nose and throat; profuse, acrid and hot discharge; much run-down condition and much weakness, sleepiness, and eyes, nose and throat being simultaneously affected.

Ipecac 30

It is specially suitable when there is vomiting and nausea, profuse mucus discharge and excessive sneezing.

Kali Bich 6

Helpful in case of pain in throat; sticky, adhering and stringy mucus which is difficult to detach and thick and purulent phlegm.

Chronic Stage

Untreated acute cases of cold, frequently inhaling dust or irritating vapours or other irritants; repeated catarrhal attacks, syphilis, etc., may lead to chronic complication.

Lyco 30

It is useful in atrophic stage when the patient has to breathe through nose, due to blocking of both the nostrils at night.

Sticta 30

Dry cough aggravation during inspiration, desire to blow the nose constantly due to atrophy thereof but no relief, nose stuffed and blocked, nostrils dry and scabs form in them can be cured by this medicine.

Puls 30

In case nasal discharge is green, yellow and foetid due to repeated catarrhal in acute form and it aggravates in warm rooms and ameliorates in cold and open places and the sense of smell and taste is lost, use of Puls 30 often helps.

Kali Sulph 3X

If after the use of Puls, throat infection develops or when Puls fails, it is a useful remedy.

Kali Iod 6

Its symptoms generally tally with those of *Kali Bich* but is more suited to syphilitic cases where there is abuse of mercury; ulceration in the nostrils, discharge is foetid, yellow or greenish black.

Mother tincture of homeopathy should be given in acute as well as chronic stages.

Blata Orient-Q

Give 5-6 drops in water, either just before the appearance of symptoms on the outset or even during the attack. It will shorten the asthmatic attack's duration and give relief. If there is asthma with bronchitis, cough with laboured breathing, and if mucus resembles pus it should be administered. Suited best to robust, stout and obese persons. Stop its use when improvement is seen, otherwise it will cause recurrence of symptoms.

Senega-Q

Give 5-6 drops in water when *Ipecac 30, Ars ALB 30* or *Lobelia* have failed to yield results. It is best when dry cough is followed by cough with excessive expectoration, sneezing, wheezing sound and pain and sense of constriction in the chest, rattling noise in chest, loss of voice, (on suddenly getting up during a rest and while moving in open air), when sweat appears and when head is lowered. Also useful in case of unsteady voice, partial paralysis of vocal cords, sore chest walls, profuse mucus, difficulty in breathing, feeling as if lungs were forced back to spine and when cough ends up in a sneeze.

Eridictyon-Q or 3X

Asthma relieved by expectoration. Bronchial pthisis, with night sweats and emaciation, cough after influenza; wheezing sounds; coryza; dull pain in right lung. Appetite poor and defective digestion. Whooping cough symptoms.

Give 5-20 drops in water, according to severity of symptoms. Avoid repeating quite often.

Lobelia Inflata-Q

In case of aggravation by any exertion, amelioration by rapid walking; feelings as if heart would stop beating; sensation of weight and pressure on the chest; asthmatic attacks leading to much weakness, ringing cough and short breath, this medicine proves useful.

Note: Choose any one or two remedies according to your symptoms and take three times a day. In case of any confusion, Please consult an experienced and well-educated homoeopathic physician.

Biochemic medicine

Bio-Plasgen No. 2

Components – Kali Phos, Magn. Phos, Nat Mur and Nat Sulph.

It is useful for nervous asthma accompanied by cough, gasping, irregular pulse, asthma with troublesome flatulence or spasms and convulsive cough with yellow sputum.

Acupressure

Massage the areas of the lungs in hands and feet with pressure, for one or two minutes, thrice a day.

Massage in the early morning, on an empty stomach.

Magnetotherapy

A pair of high power magnets should be placed under palms for 10 to 12 minutes in the morning and for the same duration in the evening, if possible (north pole under right palm and south pole under left palm). Continuous contact is necessary, without any pressure. This regulates circulatory, nervous and respiratory systems, proves beneficial in asthma and bronchitis, removes pain in chest and difficulty in breathing. If high power magnets are not available, medium power or premier magnets may be used but they are less powerful and should, therefore, be applied for 15 to 20 minutes.

The application of crescent (curved) ceramic magnet is beneficial for the troubles of nose and throat. The north pole of these magnet should be applied on the right nostril, covering the full nasal wall, for about 10 minutes, twice daily. This will gradually remove the problems of nose namely blocking, polypus, sneezing, watering, etc., and will ease the difficulty in breathing through the nose.

The crescent type ceramic magnets may able be applied on the throat, for about 10 minutes once or twice daily. This will reduce coughing, irritation, pain and other inconveniences of throat, if any.

A magnetic necklace may be worn around the neck, touching the upper part of the chest. It has proved quite effective in asthma and bronchitis. The necklace can be worn throughout the day, except while taking a bath. If one does not like to wear it during the day, one may wear it during the night.

The magnetised water prepared with high power magnets should be drunk three/four times everyday, about two ounces in each dose. The magnetised water not only removes congestion in the chest and lungs, constipation and gas formation, but also helps to regulate and improve appetite and digestion.

Colour therapy

Fill water in orange or red bottles and keep it in sunlight. Drink a cup of this water twice after consuming your food.

At night, before going to sleep, rub oil on chest, prepared by keeping oil in red bottle in the sunlight.

In winters, cover your body by orange or red saree and sit in sunrays for half an hour.

Note: Keep the water or oil in sunlight for 8 to 10 hours. Then store the bottle in an almirah, out of dust and dampness.

Treatment by Naturopathy and Yogic Exercises

Yogic exercises

Patients having cough with expectoration should be taught Dhautis which include Vamana Dhauti and Vastra Dhauti. These help in removing mucoid secretions from the stomach. Vastra Dhauti helped in the further removal of excessive mucus from the stomach.

For effective removal of sputum from the lungs, Kapalabhati Kriya (diaphragmatic breathing) is also advocated.

All these exercise should be conducted under the guidance of an experienced yoga teacher.

Exercise for relief during an attack

In a kneeling position, with arms and head resting on a table or a chair, breathe out slowly. Then let the abdomen relax and make sure the air enters the chest without any effort. Let the shoulders and chest relax. Do this slowly, otherwise it would cause wheezing.

The following are some of the important points to be particularly observed while doing an exercise:

1. Clear the nose and breathe in through the nose, and breathe out through the mouth with a whistling or hissing sound.

2. While breathing in, keep the upper chest still, so that breathing is performed by diaphragm.

3. When breathing out, the whole chest should relax.

4. All the exercise should be performed slowly without tiring the muscles.

5. The exercise may be repeated many times a day, so that the habit becomes second nature.

Expiration-inspiration ratio

The time taken for inspiration and expiration is very important for an asthma patient. Generally speaking, expiration should be longer than inspiration and in the ratio of 3:2 approximately. This applies during both rest and exertion of any kind. Speed is relatively unimportant. The patient should try to fit this rhythm to the rate at which he is breathing. When he is breathless, he should breathe within his wheeze. Any attempt to force expiration will only increase the wheeze and the spasm. He should do gentle, quick breathing with a longer expiration, while gradually reducing the speed. Breathing exercises can be learnt by the asthma patient within three to six weeks. If he likes, he can do them himself or learn from a physiotherapist or a yoga teacher.

Breathing exercise

Breathing with rhythm

Sit cross-legged on the ground or on a chair or stand with folded hands as in prayer. Keep mouth closed and breathe in through the nostrils counting one to four. Hold your breath till you count from five to eight. Start to breathe out. While breathing out count once again from one to four, hold your breath till you count from five to eight before you start inhaling. Repeat this a few more times. Increase the number of counts while breathing in and out and in between, gradually from day-to-day, to draw in more oxygen and expel more carbon dioxide.

Cleansing pranayama

Sit cross-legged on the ground or on a chair with the spine erect and muscles relaxed. Cover the right nostril with the thumb and inhale through the left nostril. Cover the left nostril too with the index finger and hold your breath for one to two counts. Release the thumb and exhale through the right nostril. Repeat this with the left nostril. Cover the left nostril with the index finger and inhale through the right. Close both the nostrils and hold for one or two counts and then exhale through the left nostril, releasing the index finger. With regular practice, the number of counts while holding the breath should increase.

This exercise corrects the disorders of the nasal cavity and lungs. The good supply of oxygen helps to purify the lungs. Those who suffer from blood pressure must not hold the breath. They can simply inhale and exhale.

Naturopathy in asthma

Naturopathy is a preventive, curative and corrective therapy with no side effects, when the rules are fully adhered to. All the methods have patient-compliance, are cost effective and easy to perform. Whenever naturopathy is tried, first of all, bowels should be cleared by purging out faecal matter from the intestines.

Taking an enema

Take a vessel, filled it with 1 to 1½ litres of lukewarm water. Before taking an enema, properly check the nozzle and vessel. Disinfect both the vessel and nozzle and allow some water to flow out of the nozzle so that no air packet disturbs water flow, as trapped air can also enter the intestines along with enema water. Only hard surface should be used while lying down on the floor but ensure that buttocks remain 2 to 4 inches higher than the floor level. By doing so, you can be rest assured that water will enter through the rectum without any obstruction. The vessel should be hung at a height of 1 metre or so above your body level. Now insert the nozzle in the rectum and raise your knees a bit so as to facilitate entry of water.

Water in the intestines should be retained till the urgency to visit the toilet arises. Do not exert any pressure while defecating. The water takes some time to act on the impacted faecal matter. It would be still better if cold water is used instead of lukewarm water. When your bowels have been cleared, you may feel another urgency to empty your stomach. It is so because adherent and tough faeces take more time to soften and come out. If you continue the practice of having an enema daily, your system will automatically and slowly get back to normalcy when your system acclimatises with the new situations.

Most of the problems occurs from chronic constipation which is removed effectively by enema water. Once your stools are normal, there won't be any indigestion, flatulence, colic, acidity, eructations, or burning sensations.

Kunjal kriya

Kunjal means elephant who first drinks plenty of water in one go and then expels (vomits out) the same later on. This kriya is a part of Nature Cure and Yoga. Those who always have their chest filled with sputum, cannot respirate comfortably, suffer from asthma, and/or other respiratory and digestive problems should practise it.

Boil about 2 – 3 litres of water in a utensil and let it cool down to lukewarm temperature. Now add some salt to it. Sit on your toes on an empty stomach and drink the water until it reaches your throat or when you develop a vomiting sensation. Now vomit the entire water from your mouth by inserting your fingers in the throat so that the entire ingested quantity of water comes out. This water is of yellow colour or phlegm; taste would be either bitter or acidic or both. Sometimes it is acidic and pungent so the throat remains bitter/acidic for some time. If you feel an urgency to defecate, you should not delay because intestinal filth will be ejected through this process.

After body has been fully emptied, do not eat or drink anything; except having an apple. For lunch have *khichri* and 10 – 20 gm of clarified butter. At about 4 pm, you should have only a cup of coffee, and bland and light diet at dinner time. Cold drink and food should not be taken, at least for 24 hours.

The whole process, as detailed above, can be repeated as and when the said disorders are felt. The abdominal portion should be kept fully wrapped, avoiding fan or/and cold in any form. Frequent repetition of this process (*Kunjal Kriya*) is advised.

Hip bath

Hip bath is recommended for purging out toxins through urine. Urine is a waste product of the body and, under no condition, should the desire to pass it be suppressed or delayed beyond the retentive capacity of your bladder. Hip bath is not only beneficial in urine, kidney and other related problems but it also imparts soothing and salutary effect on the entire abdominal area, urinary passage, kidneys, etc. It will ensure free and uninterrupted flow of urine, remove burning sensation, hesitancy, strangury, pain, etc.

Take a tub which has one end raised up. You should sit in the tub in such a way that your head rests on the raised portion of tub and your feet are placed on a stool which should be kept near, but outside, the tub so that you will be sitting in a semi-reclined position. Before you sit in the tub, make sure that water in the tub is sufficient to touch your navel. Rub your abdomen with a rough towel, from right to left, while you are sitting in the tub, but do not rub so harshly or apply hard pressure that your skin starts aching. There is no hard-and-fast rule as to the duration of hip-bath which should be any where between 10 to 20 minutes, depending on the ailment, basic structure of a person and his capacity to sit in one position. Body should be rubbed for 4 to 7 minutes or more if you can or need be.

Initially hip bath can be taken for a short time, say 2 to 4 minutes, gradually increasing the duration. During winter, reduce the duration and rub your body vigorously to warm up the body before taking your normal bath which can be had 2–3 hours after a hip bath.

Sun bath

Sun is the motivator and promoter of life. In zodiac signs, sun is the lord of all other planets and moon is accorded the status of a mother. It is a common knowledge that all other planets and stars derive their energy from the sun including the moon.

Bathing is not merely a ritual, it is our hygienic necessity also. In the western world, sun bath has primarily a cosmetic value, though they do not deny its therapeutic utility. In India, bathing has been attached with religious rituals also, as it is not only a means to body-hygiene, but also it is an exercise in itself.

As far as sun bath is concerned, it can be divided into following methods:

1. Take off your clothes or keep only the bare minimum on the body so that maximum part is exposed to sunrays.

2. Keep a bucketful of water under the sun and take bath only after the water has warmed up.

3. Take bath in the open with warm water under the sun.

4. Massage the whole body with mustard oil under the sun and thereafter take a bath with water which has been warmed under sunrays.

All the four mentioned facts can be summed up and joined together to derive maximum advantage from sun bath. While you expose your body to sunrays, you should vigorously massage your whole body with mustard oil. After massage, your body will get exposed to sunrays for at least 30 to 40 minutes. But, before you start to massage your body under the sun, keep a bucketful of water exposed to direct sunrays so that, when you have finished your oil massage, water, (to be used for talking bath) is ready in good time, or at least ready upto the time you have massaged your body.

Enjoy sun bath in the open but, when cold winds are blowing and sunrays are also not so hot as to charge your body with heat, it is better to first wrap your body and then sit in the sun. Exposure to cold must be ruled out under any circumstances. Sun bath opens the clogged pores of your skin, by means of sweat, which is indicative of the activity of sweat glands. If your body fails to sweat it out, sip hot water to induce sweating. Even putting on woollen clothes and sitting in the sun would suffice to induce proper sweating. By nature, certain people habitually sweat more than others but, in such a case, sweat need not be wiped, rather it may be allowed to have its own course or, if there is more sweat due to oil massage or excessive heat of sun, sweat should be absorbed into the body along with oil.

Never take a bath with cold water after sun bath, but always use hot or lukewarm water. Sun bath would yield better and quicker results if taken between 10 am and 12 noon. Health status must be taken into active consideration while deciding to have a sun bath, as wrong choice or decision is likely to cause more harm than good.

Fasting

Fasting does not mean total abstention from food. In fact, process of fasting has been devised to rectify the ravages and upsets caused by irregular overeating or when the needs of the body and health are relegated or subjugated to avarice of palate. Let it be clearly understood that very few people die due to not eating enough, whereas millions die of overeating. When food is deeply fried with saturated fats, enriched with spices, meats, (excluding essential nutrients), there should be no doubt about imbibing disease.

When body is treated like a dust-bin, food relaxations and indiscretions are treated as normal episodes, when everything and anything finds its way into our stomach, we must not expect metabolism to work better. Overeating is a major cause for onset of acidity, flatulency, colic, burning sensation, loose motions or constipated bowels, rise in cholesterol level, diabetes, respiratory disorders, cardiac disorders, joint pains, gout, arthritis, high blood pressure to name a few only. Too much consumption of alcohol, fats, tobacco, spices, fast food, etc., are sufficient to cause multiple health hazards.

Kinds of fasting

- Complete fast
- Partial fast
- Fast on fruits only
- Fast on fruits and vegetables only
- Fast on milk and banana diet
- Fast on milk and mango
- Fast on honey and lemon
- Giving up one food item each day
- Fasting on water alone

Fast in a way to cleanse the body and remove the obnoxious and harmful toxins. Fast is a protective device, if taken in health, but will prove a curative and preventive device, if taken during a disease.

Note: Please consult a good physician before fasting in such cases.

Following persons should not take to fasting

- Young and growing children
- Pregnant and lactating ladies
- Old, infirm and bed-ridden person
- Those who suffer from malnutrition
- Economically weaker persons, labourers, and travellers poor persons
- Women during menstrual periods or menopause or during puberty
- Persons with low glucose level in the blood
- Any cardiac disease/low-blood pressure patients
- Persons suffering any acute illness

How to begin

Those who are gluttons, have sedentary habits, who like overeating, lead an easy and luxurious life, are addicts, do not do any physical activity, can initially, face plenty of problems if they take to fasting. Such person should start with partial fasting, that is, they should miss one meal. When they succeed in the first venture, they can switch on to a complete fast but, for the type of persons categorised here, it is not easy to fast for the whole day. Fasting is another way of sacrificing, because during fast you have forego a food item or a meal which you love most.

Fasting not only purifies your body but also purifies and elevates your mental and intellectual faculties. It is a unique way to purge out impurities from your word, deed and mind. It elevates your good and noble traits but, at the same time, improves your general approach to life.

Fasting balances various juices and enzymes, apart from secretions/excretions, within the body so as to favour and improve the general metabolism of the body, finally leading to a normal health. If the beginners experience any disorder or discomfort during fasting, they should, at once, seek guidance of a naturopath. As a first step, reduce food quantity from your diet, either skip breakfast or lunch or dinner. When no problem is encountered by sacrificing one meal (for 7 days), add to it one more meal (to be missed), and finally you will reach a situation when, even giving up whole day's meals will not pose any problem.

When you end your fast, take a very light diet at night: a glass full of milk, 1 – 2 pieces of seasonal fruits, 1 – 2 buttered slices. Beverages may be used hot, cold or lukewarm, according to the weather conditions or better still what suits you best. If the aspirant's aim is to overload the stomach at the end of the fast, it is better if he does not opt for fasting, as fasting is no occasion for overeating or satiating your taste buds.

Ideal fast

An ideal fast is that in which there is no fatigue, run-down conditions, weakness, loss of appetite, loose motions or constipation, fever, etc. Natural appetite, general resistance and strength of the body, downward trend of various disorders, regulated respiration and circulation, reduction in pains and aches, cheerfulness, elevation of spirits, renewed energy, etc., are some of the benefits which should follow a successful fast.

If a fast is kept for the whole day, one should take some honey and lemon juice to avoid weakness, fatigue and longing for food. During summer, one must not stay without the intake of water, or else electrolytic balance will get disturbed. To avoid dehydration, mix a juice of a lemon and a pinch of salt and a teaspoon of sugar to a glassful of water which can be sipped or drunk as and when needed. The diabetics can substitute sugar with a teaspoon of honey. If you take either of the recipes, detailed above, you are not likely to feel weak or run the risk of dehydration.

Fast on milk, banana or seasonal fruits

This will form part of partial fast when, at the time of breakfast, a glass of milk with two bananas or one/two pieces of some seasonal fruits are taken. It will suffice to meet food requirements for a normal person, for about 6 – 8 hours but, in between honey, lemon juice with water, may be taken. During summer some persons prefer a glass of whey or 250 gm of curd, to which a piece of banana or any other fresh fruit may be added. It is advised that ailing persons should never take to fasting, unless they have been specifically advised by their attending physicians/naturopaths.

Household remedies of asthma

Include figs, grapes, dates, papayas and apples in the diet. Take any of these fruits during breakfast regularly for a few days.

One teaspoon juice of tulsi leaves, ginger, onion and honey should be mixed. Take this mixture twice daily for one month at a stretch. Prepare a fresh mixture every time.

Take fresh unboiled cow's milk twice a day, that is, in the morning and at bed time. Those having low tolerance to raw milk, should avoid taking it unboiled. Instead, they have milk boiled with garlic.

One piece of ginger and three garlic cloves should be boiled in water for five minutes and this solution should be sipped steaming hot.

Treatment by Allopathy

Asthma has two components: the spasm and the swelling.

The acute phase of the disease is characterised by bronchospasm.

Asthmatic patients have hyper-responsive airways which swell in response to inflammatory cells and chemicals mediators. The epithelial lining of their airways, sheds, leaving behind a damaged surface. The shed cells combine with mucus and eosinophils to form tenacious plugs, which block the airways. In addition to this, there is oedema of the bronchial wall with smooth muscle contraction and hypertrophy. These aspects broadly constitute the swelling components of asthma.

Thus, the spasm and the swelling together lead to bronchial obstruction in asthma. And this gives rise to the twin aspects of asthma treatment, relief and prevention – relieving the spasm and preventing the swelling.

Anti-asthma drugs are classified into relievers and preventers.

What are relievers?

Relievers are broncho-dilators which relieve acute bronchospasm by relaxing the bronchial smooth muscles. These drugs have no role in the management the inflammation but give immediate relief during acute attacks. These are effective for 4 to 6 hours and generally used in conjunction with preventers.

How do they act?

Reliever drugs cause bronchodilation and thus give immediate relief. But inflammation change, and may, in fact increase if only relievers are used.

Commonly used reliever drugs

- Short-acting Beta2-agonists-salbutamol, terbutaline
- Anticholinergics-Ipratropium bromide
- Short-acting theophylline
- Adrenaline injections

What are preventers?

Preventer drugs help to prevent acute attacks of bronchospasm and reduce their frequency by controlling the underlying inflammation. These drugs however do not give immediate relief from symptoms. In fact, the onset of action may take up to three hours. However, their duration of action is long. These are used on a long-term basis to control symptoms and underlying inflammation.

How do they act?

Preventers are used over a long period to control the underlying inflammation. At an early stage, preventers can almost normalise the inflammation in the airways, thus controlling the disease.

Commonly used preventer drugs

- *Corticosteroids*

Inhaled: Beclomethasone dipropionate, Budesonide, Fluticasone propionate, Oral/Parenteral, Prednisolone/ Methylpred-nisolone, Dexamethasone, Hydrocortisone

- *Mast Cell Stabiliser Inhaled:* Sodium cromoglycate
- *Long-acting b-agonists Inhaled:* Salmeterol Oral: sustained-release salbutamol/Terbutaline
- Long-acting theophyllines
- Ketotifen

Among the above, the most potent anti-inflammatory agents are the corticosteriods.

Mode of medication

- Inhalation
- Oral
- Parenteral

Currently the most favoured route worldwide is inhalation.

Logic of the inhaled route

In the treatment of asthma, the target site is the tracheobronchial tree. It is thus logical to inhale the drug as it is delivered directly to the lungs. With this direct delivery, one can expect rapid action with much smaller doses and hence lesser side effects. On the other hand, through the oral or parenteral route the drug reaches the lungs only after passing through the stomach and/or the systemic circulation, increasing the probability of side effects as shown in the figure.

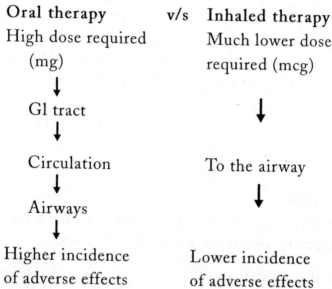

Oral therapy	v/s	Inhaled therapy
High dose required (mg)		Much lower dose required (mcg)
↓		
Gl tract		↓
↓		
Circulation		To the airway
↓		
Airways		↓
↓		
Higher incidence of adverse effects		Lower incidence of adverse effects

Inhaled steroids vs oral steroids

Studies show that 1.5 to 2 mg (1500-2000 mcg) of inhaled steroid has beneficial effect similar to 30 to 40 mg of prednisone (oral steroid).

This clearly shows that through inhalation therapy the dose required is less than 1/10th of the dose required by oral route.

Advantages of inhalation therapy
- Targeted drug delivery
- Fast onset of action
- Non-invasive
- Minimal dosage
- Reduced systemic side effects
- Avoids GI irritation (as compared to oral route)
- Avoids pain, irritation and/or muscle damage (as encountered with parenteral formulations)

What is a DPI?
A dry powder inhaler (DPI), uses the drug in a dry powder form. The device commercially available for this purpose is the Rotahaler which uses Rotacaps, or gelatin capsules containing the drug in the powder form. This rotacap is inserted into the Rotahaler, which is then manipulated to separate the capsule halves and release the powder. When the patient inhales from the mouthpiece of the Rotahaler, the medicine is directly breathed into the lungs.

Difference between DPI and MDI
The dry powders and their delivery devices were invented as it was found that a large number of patients had difficulty in using the conventional metered dose inhaler (MDI).

This was primarily because of the following reasons:
- Patients could not synchronise the MDI with inspiration.
- Faulty techniques led to decreased drug delivery resulting in poor control of symptoms. Consequently, discontinuation of therapy was common.
- MDI use CFCs (chlorofluoro-carbons) as a liquid propellant. They are considered to be unfriendly to the environment because they damage the ozone layer, a phenomenon which increases exposure to ultraviolet radiation. This created a need for propellant free inhaler devices such as DPIs.

Advantages of DPI
- Being a breath-activated device, it eliminates the need for coordination of inspiration with drug delivery.
- DPI is simple to use. The physicians can easily train patients within minutes. This saves precious time for busy practitioners.
- It is small and can be easily carried by the patients.
- DPI is suitable for use in almost all patient group, except for those less than 4 years of age. It can be easily used even by arthritic patients who have difficulty in coordinating the actuation with inspiration.
- Studies suggest that patients more easily accept the DPI, since they can readily identify with capsules (Rotacaps).

- The cost initiation of therapy with DPI is relatively less.
- Only one device has to be purchased for administering various drugs.

Peak flow meter

A peak flow meter can be used at a clinic or at home to measure how well a person is breathing.

- It helps the doctor decide if someone has asthma.
- It helps to see how bad an asthma attack is.
- It also helps the doctor see how well asthma is controlled over time.

If a peak flow meter is used every day at home, the patient can anticipate possible breathing problems before the wheezing and coughing starts. The patient can thus take prophylactic doses of medicine.

There are many kinds of peak flow meters.

How to Use a Peak Flow Meter

- Slide the little marker down as far as it will go. This sets the meter to zero.
- Stand up. Take a big breath with your mouth open. Hold the meter in one hand. Keep your fingers away from the numbers.
- Quickly close your mouth firmly around the tube. Do not put your tongue in the hole. Blow once as fast and hard as you can.
- The marker will go up and stay there. Do not touch the marker.
- Note the number on a piece of paper or on a chart.

- Blow two more times. Push the button down each time. Write the number down each time.

How to use a peak flow chart at home

- Find your peak flow number in the morning and evening.
- Each morning and each evening blow three times into the meter.
- After each blow, mark the spot where the marker stopped.
- Put the meter next to peak flow chart to help you find the spot to mark.
- Circle the highest of the three numbers. That is your peak flow number.

Diet

Proper diet taken at regular times is very important for a patient of asthma. This not only prevents attacks from occurring but also lessens the severity.

The diet should be light, nutritious and well balanced. It should not contain items which the patient is not comfortable with. For instance, North Indians feel that rice taken at night causes discomfort in breathing. This may be due to the fact that to satisfy hunger with rice, one has to take a large quantity of it, which bloats the stomach and thus hinders the full and proper working of the diaphragm for respiration. Edibles, that patients are not comfortable with, should be avoided. These can range from fruits such as bananas, to vegetables such as lady's finger, to lentils such as *urad* (black gram). For some, cold drinks and sour preparations like sauces and pickles provoke coughing and are to be avoided. Generally, spices should be avoided in one's diet.

Asthma patients should not have overeat. Fullness of the stomach after meals – in particular at night, causes discomfort in breathing and can precipitate breathlessness. Many small meals should be taken instead of a large one. Fried food should be avoided as far as possible and sweets should not be eaten at night. A patient of asthma will notice that he feels more comfortable during the night if his stomach is not heavy. So dinner should be taken at least two hours before going to sleep.

Asthma patients should take more of fruits, vegetables, cheese, eggs, chicken. But all of these should be taken in moderation. Adequate variety in the diet is to be provided, so that the patient does not get bored.

Asthma patient should avoid fried and rich food.

Diet for children

Children who develop asthma have an inability to correct weight imbalances. Overweight children are hence unable to shed weight and underweight ones are unable to gain weight. Accordingly, special attention has to be given to their diet.

A child requires more calories per kilogram of body weight than an adult, because his basic metabolic rate is higher and more calories are needed by the child for growth. An asthmatic child has an even greater metabolic rate because of hurried breathing.

Such a child needs extra carbohydrates and proteins. If the diet is otherwise well balanced, extra addition of minerals and vitamins are unnecessary.

A liberal amount of water should be given to children because they lose a lot of it in respiration. Meal hours should be regular and as far as possible, nibbling between meals should not be allowed.

A child should not be allowed to eat certain foods, for example, pickles and sauces. On the other hand, a child's likes and dislikes should be anticipated and variety introduced in a well-balanced diet. The child should not be forced to eat the foods he/she dislikes.

If the child is otherwise healthy – eating, playing and sleeping well, but not eating enough according to the parents' standard, then it is parent and not the child who needs to be instructed.

While some children like to live disciplined lives, others don't. There are some children who find drinking milk everyday monotonous; such children should be offered various milk products.

It should be borne in mind that a diet rich in sweets, while providing adequate calories, could still be quite deficient in protein content.

School-going children often hurry through their breakfast because they get up late and then hurry through their lunch because they have to play. They end up eating a heavy dinner, which is wrong. A full stomach while going to bed is more liable to lead to an attack of asthma during the night.

Diet for the aged
The lessened activity and lowered metabolic rate in the elderly, means that they require fewer calories.

If the patient is also suffering from some other disease like arthritis or angina, activity is further reduced.

If the person is taking corticosteroids, whether occasionally or regularly, then old age plus the effect of these drugs, leads to weakening of the bones (osteoporosis) because of deficiency of calcium, proteins, vitamins, minerals and hormones. It is not uncommon to find in an X-ray of the chest that one or more of the vertebrae are broken and collapsed. The whole body of an older asthmatic shrinks in height, in musculature and in girth.

If the patient has lost weight, the calorific content of the diet should be increased, making the patient feel better.

The patient must be asked to take more proteins, milk, cheese, pulses, soyabeans; if non-vegetarian, the patient can have chicken or its soup, meat, egg and fish provided he or she, is not allergic to any of these. For the sake of variety in diet, custard pudding can be taken, particularly if mastication is a problem because of loss of teeth.

Intake of fat should be limited. Suitable multivitamin tablets with mineral should be added to the daily diet.

Injections of an anabolic steroid is helpful in older people for protein retention and will lead to an increase in weight and a general feeling of being energised. A decadurabolin injection I/m once a fortnight has been found to be helpful.

Mixed Diet	Vegetarian
On Rising	
A glass of warm water, light tea – one cup	A glass of warm water light tea – one cup
Breakfast	
Egg, half-boiled or scrambled, buttered toast, seasonal fruits	Porridge or cornflakes with milk and sugar, toast and butter, seasonal fruits
11 am	
Fruit juice (Orange) – 1 cup	Fruit juice (Orange) – 1 cup
Lunch	
Meat or chicken with boiled potatoes and beans/seasonal vegetables *Chappatis* (cereal) Custard – ½ cup	Curd – 1 cup Lentils – 1 cup Cooked vegetables *Chappatis* (cereal) Custard – ½ cup
4 pm	
Tea with biscuits	Tea with biscuits or lightly fried cheese
Dinner	
Cooked vegetables Dal *Chappatis* (cereal)	Cooked vegetables Dal *Chappatis* (cereal)

Avoid

- Fried and fatty foods
- Overloading your stomach
- Smoking
- Drinking
- Sweet dish at night
- Going out after dinner on cold nights and exposure to cold air

Prefer

- Eat simple food, without spices, at regular hours
- Take light and nourishing food to which one is not allergic
- Take plenty of water during an attack of asthma
- Take dinner early in the evening, two hours before sleep
- Take a very light dinner so that the stomach is almost empty when it is time to sleep

Frequently Asked Questions

Are there any tests to determine the inflammation of the airways?

Yes, assessment of airway inflammation is usually possible by clinical symptoms and signs. Peak flow rates and lung function tests usually confirm the clinical findings and are helpful in diagnosing and monitoring the disease. To assess the presence of airway inflammation, the following tests can be done:

 i)   Sputum eosinophil counts
 ii) Bronchial biopsies or bronchoalveolar lavage
 iii) Serum eosinophilic cationic protein levels
 iv) Exhaled nitric oxide

As mentioned earlier, these tests are not commonly performed in clinical practice at all, and are usually reserved for research purposes and clinical trials to assess the anti-inflammatory effects or certain drugs.

What is spirometry/pulmonary function tests?
This denotes recording airflow obstruction: airflow obstruction can be measured with the help of minipeak flow meters. This instrument provides a cheap and

reliable method of measuring airflow obstruction and allows the patients to objectively assess the control of their asthma and its response to treatment. Acute episodes of asthma are mostly preceded by a gradual deterioration in control and this may not be apparent otherwise but may be detected by peak flow meter recordings.

Name the agents of occupational asthma.

Chemicals
- Isocyanide
- Hair sprays
- Aluminium
- Platinum salts
- Nickel
- Tungsten carbide
- Colophony
- Formaldehyde

Enzymes
- Bacillus subtills
- Trypsin

Animals
- Rodents
- Shellfish
- Larger mammals
- Locusts

Vegetable sources
- Wood dusts
- Grains
- Cotton, hemp and flax
- Gum acacia and tragacanth
- Coffee beans
- Tea leaves
- Cotton seeds

Drugs
- Penicillin
- Salbutamol
- Piperazine
- Pesticides/insecticides may also cause occupational asthma

What are the hazards of long term oral steroid therapy?

Though oral steroid therapy is often required to control acute and severe asthma for short periods, long-term administration though effective is extremely harmful. The important hazards of long-term therapy include:

   i) Hypertension
  ii) Osteoporosis
 iii) Hypothalamic-pituitary adrenal axis suppression
  iv) Diabetes
   v) Cataract
  vi) Obesity

vii) Skin thinning (easy bruisability)

viii) Muscle weakness recommended when oral steroids are considered for patients with

- Tuberculosis
- Parasitic infections
- Osteoporosis
- Glaucoma
- Diabetes
- Severe depression
- Peptic ulcers

What are the goals of asthma management in adults?

The goals of long-term asthma management in adults are as follows:

i) Minimal symptoms, including nighttime symptoms.

ii) Minimal asthma episodes or attacks.

iii) No emergency visits to doctors or hospitals.

iv) Minimal need for as needed (quick relief) B2-agonist therapy.

v) No limitations on physical activities, including running and other exercises.

vi) Minimal side effects from drugs.

Should preventive therapy for adult-onset asthma be given life long?

Just like patients with hypertension and diabetes, asthmatics also require daily medication to prevent attacks, life-long. Usually, the lowest possible dose of inhaled corticosteroid that controls symptoms would be sufficient.

If the patient insists on stopping the therapy because he feels well and refuses to listen to his physicians advice he/she will invariably return with earlier symptoms.

How does one start preventive therapy in adults?
This should be done with either oral steroids or high-dose inhaled steroids. When starting with low-dose inhaled steroids, one can face many problems. As inhaled steroids have a slow onset of action, patients who are not controlled, lose confidence in the treatment and this is likely to decrease compliance. It is therefore more sensible to start at a higher dose (800 – 1600 mcg/day) which will be effective and then reduce to the minimal dose needed to maintain control. In patients with more severe wheezing, even a short course of oral steroids can be started along with the inhaled steroids.

What are the usual maintenance doses of inhaled steroids in adults?
To put it simply, the maintenance dose is that which controls the symptoms of the patients on a regular basis. This can be highly individualised. The lowest maintenance doses in adults of beclomethasone and budesonide is 400 mcg/day. In some instances, patients have been maintained on doses as low as 200 mcg/day or budesonide.

Once asthma control is achieved, should the dose of inhaled steroids be increased or decreased?

Once asthma control is achieved, the primary objective should be to reduce and omit oral steroids if these had been instituted. Thereafter, if control is sustained for at least 3 months, a gradual reduction in the dose of inhaled steroids may be possible.

If control is not achieved, one may have to consider stepping up treatment. Always check:

- Control inhalation technique
- Compliance
- Allergen avoidance/avoidance of trigger factors

At what frequency should the dose of inhaled steroids be reduced?

Always remember that patients deteriorate differently when the dose of inhaled steroids is reduced. Therefore, always reduce the dose gradually.

The views of an expert panel report were that the dose of inhaled corticosteroids may be reduced about 25 per cent every two to three months to the lowest possible dose required to maintain control.

Can inhaled steroids causes side effects?

In general, inhaled corticosteroids are well tolerated and safe at the recommended dosages. However a few adverse effects may be noted and their management is briefly discussed as follows:

Oral candidiasis

Reduce the frequency of dosing: use topical/oral antifungal agents.

Dysphonia

Temporary reduction in dosage and voice rest.

Reflex cough and bronchospasm

Slow down the rate of inspiration, pre-treatment with an inhaled B2-agonist.

Osteoporosis

In patients at risk (especially elderly females), concurrent calcium supplements and vitamin D (qestrogen replacement where appropriate) is reasonable.

In high doses for prolonged periods in the elderly, skin thinning and easy bruisability, cataracts and impaired glucose metabolism have occasionally been noted.

How can side effects from inhaled steroids be prevented?

Side effects from inhaled steroids are rare and to prevent even these from occurring, there are various methods that help immensely to reduce oropharyngeal deposition and subsequent local and systematic side effect.

Some Objective Questions

Could you be a potential asthmatic?

	Yes	No
1. Is there a history of asthma in the family?	☐	☐
2. Do you have coughing problem at the change of season?	☐	☐
3. Do you have bouts of sneezing at the change of season?	☐	☐
4. Do you often have throat infection?	☐	☐
5. Do you get breathlessness after exertion during the change of season?	☐	☐
6. Do you have breathing problems when it is windy?	☐	☐
7. Do you work/live in a polluted environment?	☐	☐

The more 'Yes' you have, the more chances you have of having asthma.

Is your cough allergic in nature?

	Yes	No

1. Does the cough occur in a particular season or at change of season?

    ☐   ☐

2. Is the cough aggravated in a particular season or at change of season?

    ☐   ☐

3. Is it accompanied with bouts of sneezing as well?

    ☐   ☐

4. Is this coughing more at night than during the day time?

    ☐   ☐

5. Did you have ezcema in your childhood?

    ☐   ☐

6. Is there history of bouts of sneezing, eczema or coughing in the family, that is, parents and siblings?

    ☐   ☐

If the answer to even two of the above questions is in the affirmative, the cough is allergic in nature.

Are the child's symptoms due to asthma ?

	Yes	No

1. Is the child prone to frequently bouts of coughing?

    ☐   ☐

2. Does the child frequently have a running of the nose?

    ☐   ☐

3. Are the child's coughing episodes, sometimes followed by fever?

    ☐   ☐

4. Has the child a wheeze in the chest? This can be ascertained by putting your ear against his or her chest.

    ☐   ☐

5. Has the child ever developed an oozing rash on the face?

    ☐   ☐

6. Does the child, or did the child, get abdominal colic at any time?

    ☐   ☐

The more the 'Yes' answers, the greater is the likelihood that your child actually does suffer from asthma.

Dos and Don'ts

Dos

- Get up in the morning at a regular hour.
- Take morning walks or do some other physical exercise.
- Take a simple diet, without spices, at regular hours. Discretion in diet should be strictly observed.

- Keep your bedroom clean of dust. It should have no rugs or carpets in it.
- Take your medicine regularly as directed by your doctor.
- Always maintain regularity in your daily work routine.
- Always sleep early at night at regular hours.

Don'ts

- Do not disturb the physical as well as mental activities of your daily routine.
- Try to avoid smoking completely.
- Hard drinks should be avoided.
- Do not overeat as it triggers asthma attack.
- Keep yourself away from smoke and dust.
- Keep your room pollution free.

Enlarged Tonsils and Asthma

Tonsils stand like two sentinels on either side of the pharynx, the middle portion of the throat. They defend the body against germs or other dangerous substances that try to enter our body through the mouth or nose. They trap these germs inside their structure and then with the help of lymphatic cells, of which the tonsils are made of, provide protective antibodies. These antibodies circulate in the blood and fight those intruders which somehow manage to bypass the tonsils. The antibody forming tissue is present in the other parts of the body also, but in the shape of the tonsils, it forms the first line of defence of the body.

During childhood, the body is exposed to many germs for the first time, and needs to be protected against them. In this process, the tonsils work vigorously and in some children get unduly enlarged.

Whether the enlarged tonsil should be removed or not is a controversial question; still more controversial is whether the tonsils should be removed in a child who has some allergic manifestations such as cough and wheeze. There are three different views available on the subject:

- Tonsils act initially as the site and subsequently as the source of infection in the body. Their removal would favourably influence the course of asthma or even prevent its occurrence in a susceptible individual.
- Tonsils perform an important function in preventing the spread of infection from the nose and throat into the bronchi and the lungs. Their removal, therefore, would lead to a mild asthma developing into a severe one or might even precipitate asthma in a susceptible individual.
- The presence or the removal of tonsils makes no difference to the allergic state of an individual. The removal of tonsils can, therefore, neither prevent asthma nor precipitate its onset.

Allergic children are, no doubt, more susceptible to infections, particularly those of the throat and if the infection is localised in the tonsils and appears again and again, the tonsils may need to be removed. But the removal should be done with the understanding that it may have an effect upon the asthma. At best, the removal of an infected tonsils may do away with one factor which may, indirectly, have something to do with the aggravation or precipitation of asthma, but it will not touch the basic factor of allergy in the child. Until this is investigated and tackled properly, symptoms of asthma will continue to appear. A comparative study of asthmatic children whose tonsils had been removed and those in whom they were allowed to remain, showed no statistical difference in the severity of the symptoms of asthma. Both the groups showed the same percentage of mild, moderate and severe case.

Even those who advocate that surgical removal of the tonsils (tonsillectomy) in asthma patients proves useful, agree that the benefits derived from tonsillectomy are greater in the first post-operative year than in the second. If tonsils are the cause of trouble, one would expect improvement.

An asthmatic child with merely enlarged tonsils needs to be investigated for allergy on the same lines as any other asthmatic patient. The cause of allergy, whether inhalant or ingestant, must be found out, and then either eliminated from the diet or submitted to proper hyposensitisation, provided the child is cooperative.

Perennial Sneezing or Allergic Rhinitis

Some patients have sneezing and a running nose almost all the year round.

Symptoms

A majority of them complain of a blocked or stuffy nose and of post-nasal discharge as well. Many of them snore at night because of this condition, and develop the habit of breathing through the mouth. They experience discomfort in the ears as well due to a blocking of the ear tubes, called eustachian tubes, that connect the ear to the throat.

Children develop a peculiar mannerism of wiping their nose, as they elevate the tip of the nose with the palm of the hand and wriggle the nose and mouth from side to side. This gives them a temporary relief from the symptoms. Constant rubbing of the nose sometimes leads to the development of a crease across the nose, called the 'allergic crease'. The mucous membranes of the paranasal sinuses may also be involved in the allergic process and infections, causing blockage of the opening of the sinuses and accumulation of the secretions; there may be associated fever. The middle ear may get infected repeatedly, causing flow of pus from the ears. Some of the patients develop cough and wheezing as well.

Exposure to cold wind, sunlight, dust and fumes and such causes, precipitate the onset of symptoms or aggravate them. These symptoms occur more often in the early morning, but may last throughout the day and even the night.

Examination of the nose

In the acute stage, examination of the nose, reveals a swollen, greyish-pale mucous membrane which is covered over with mucus secretion, the swollen mucous membrane may even be obstructing the nasal passages.

In the chronic stage of the disease, the nasal membrane may be swollen, baggy and pearl grey, with mucus and pus or even frank pus, if there is a superimposed infection. Nasal polyps, which look like a bunch of grapes hanging from the mucous membrane, may be seen blocking passages in the nose.

Diagnosis

While diagnosis of the condition is assisted by the history of the disease, a family history of allergy, and examination of the nose, more important, is the laboratory examination of nasal secretion for a large count of eosinophil cells – a type of white blood cell, which, on staining, takes on a red colour, indicative of allergy.

But all this gives no indication of the agents to which the patient is allergic. This needs skin testing with the different possible allergens such as pollen and dust.

Treatment

Exposure to likely allergens, pollutants and irritants must be reduced. These include house dust, outside dust and airborne particulate matter from workplace situations. Strong fumes whether from the kitchen or the laboratory or strong perfumes should be avoided.

After the causative allergens have been found, hyposensitization is the best method of treatment. The results, however, are not as good as in the case of seasonal sneezing or hay fever.

In the circumstances where arrangements for hyposensitization are not available or till such time as the effect of hyposensitization does not appear, drug treatment has to be given to provide relief from symptoms. Antihistamines help, but not as much as in seasonal cases. Nose drops containing ephedrine and antihistamines also give temporary relief; care must, however, be taken to limit their use to the minimum. Nose drops containing corticosteroids have not proved very helpful. Cauterization – burning the mucous membrane so as to make it insensitive and such like measures which destroy viable (live) tissue do more harm than good. Nasal surgery is rarely, if ever, indicated.

Adequate improvement obtained after hyposensitization and drug treatment leads very often to disappearance of the nasal polyps as well; they need no surgical excision, unless they are obstructing the nose to the extent that respiration becomes difficult.

Differentiation from common cold

Frequent occurrences of the common cold, a virus infection, accompanied with additional bacterial infection, sometimes makes it difficult to differentiate it from perennial allergic rhinitis. Common cold usually begins with malaise, aches and pains, diminished appetite and a slight rise of temperature. A running nose and sneezing follow, either immediately, or soon after. The nasal discharge is at first watery, but later it becomes thick. With the nasal obstruction, a headache may develop along with the loss of the sense of taste. The obstruction of nasal passages also leads to breathing in through the mouth. The symptoms may persist for some days or even weeks.

The history of the disease, family history, examination of the nose and nasal smears help to differentiate between perennial allergic rhinitis and the common cold. A nasal smear does not show eosinophils in a viral infection, while it does so in a case of perennial allergic rhinitis. Skin tests, using a variety of allergens, also help in determining the ailment, by showing up as positive or negative skin tests against various allergens also help in differentiating the conditions.

Causes of allergy
- House dust and mites
- Plant pollens
- Fungi
- Insects/Insect bites
- Food articles
- Animals
- Changing weather conditions,
- Chemicals, paints, insecticides, pesticides, fertilizers (industrial pollution)
- Smoke and fly-ash
- Heredity

Investigations
1. Pulmonary Function Test
2. Radiological (X-Ray) examination
3. Skin hypersensitivity tests
4. Aerial blood gas analysis

Grading of skin tests
Grade, size of weal and size of redness can be determined from the following table:

Grade	Size of Weal	Size of Redness
0	Same as control	Same as control
1 + 2	times more than control	10-20 mm
2 + 3	times more than the control	20-30 mm
3 + 4	times more than the control	More than 30 mm

4 + 5	times more than the control	More than 40 mm

Normally negative reactions point out to absence of antibody against the tested allergen but other considerations (such as the use of weak, inadequate and deteriorated extracts) can account for negative reaction/absence of antibody. Skin tests are carried out for the following:

1. Grasses   -   such as sorghum, cynoden, etc.

2. Trees   -   putranjiva, cassia, eucalyptus, etc.

3. Weeds   -   ageraturm, adhatoda, asphodelons, Brassica, argemone, chenopodium, album, Xanthium, parthenium, dodonea, artemesia, amaranthus and parthenium, etc.

4. Fungi   -   candida, aspergillus fumigatus, cladodos-porium, helminthosp-orium, etc.

5. Pets   -   cat, horse, dog.

6. Dusts   -   wheat dust, house dust, paper dust, cotton dust, etc.

There are variable timings when the above mentioned allergens surface in a particular month of the year but grading remains the same in all conditions.

Premonitory symptoms

Children who have allergic symptoms are more liable to get asthma. These symptoms are

- unusual and persistent colic;
- need for frequent changes of feeding formulas;
- unexplained diarrhoea or constipation;
- extreme likes and dislikes for certain foods;
- excessive vomiting;
- unexplained skin rashes;
- discharge of pus from the ears (otitis media);

If one or both the parents have some allergic disorder, there is a likelihood that some of their children may also have it, perhaps, in the form of asthma.

Preventive measures

Special precautions are required in case of those children whose parents show certain symptoms of allergy. The child is also at the risk of getting the allergic disorder.

It has been reported that a breast-fed infant has one-seventh the chance of getting allergic eczema compared to the bottle fed baby. An early introduction of solid foods in the diet of an infant also predisposes it to allergy.

Milk should be boiled before consuming. Eggs should not be introduced in the diet before six months of age and after that only boiled eggs should be given. Unboiled eggs should never be given. The introduction of foods that are most commonly cause allergic reactions, that is, egg, wheat, fish, cocoa, etc. should be delayed.

Dust-free environments

The environment of a child who is potentially allergic is very important. The child's bedroom should be reserved as a place for sleeping, not for play. It should be kept as free as possible of inhaleable allergens. The furniture should be of a type which does not promote the presence of dust or mould spores. The mattress should be completely enclosed in tight dust-proof casing or should be made of foam rubber. Dust-collecting drapes, bedspreads and wool rugs should be avoided. Blankets should preferably be made of synthetic fibres and covered with a cotton case. The child's bed should not be placed next to an open window since a chill caused by cold weather may give rise to symptoms.

Pets should not be allowed in the bedroom and are best kept out of the house, as dogs and cats bring in dust and drop strands of fur. Stuffed toys should be kept out.

Routine cleaning, dusting, etc. should preferably be done when the child is away at school. White-washing and painting, etc. too should be done when the child is out of the house.

Protection from infection

A potentially allergic child should be immunised like any other child, against whooping cough, diphtheria, tetanus, typhoid, cholera and polio. Because so many allergic children are sensitive to eggs, vaccines containing egg protein are a special hazard to them and should be avoided. In case there is a doubt, a preliminary scratch test with the vaccine should be performed, and the vaccine should be given only once there is surety of no reaction.

Every precaution must be taken to see that the child does not get a bacterial or viral infection. But in case infection does occur, treatment must be prompt and adequate. Usually, symptoms of allergy are precipitated during such an infection.

Children predisposed to allergy are likely to do well in a dry climate, away from the seashore and, in environs free of industrial air pollutants.

Special recommendations are some times offered for pregnant mothers who are allergic. Some doctors believe that potentially allergen foods such as eggs, milk, nuts and fish should be curtailed considerably during pregnancy; others take a moderate position and allow the mother all foods but not in excessive quantities.

Postnatal care for your new born

Do's

- Preferably breastfeed your child. Chances of developing allergies is more in bottle-fed babies.
- Boil the milk properly before giving it to the baby.
- Introduction of common allergen foods such as eggs, wheat, fish, cocoa, etc. should be delayed.

- Dust-proof casing or a foam rubber mattress should be used. A dust-free environment is very important for a child.
- Keep the pets away from the baby's bedroom.
- Stuffed toys should be kept out of the crib.

Dont's

- Avoid early introduction of solid foods in the diet.
- Eggs should be avoided in the diet of a child aged below nine months.
- Thereafter, boiled eggs can be given.
- Dust collecting drapes, bedspreads, wool rugs and carpets should be avoided.

Is your cough allergic in nature?

	Yes	No
1. Does the cough occur in a particular season or at change of season?	☐	☐
2. Is the cough aggravated in a particular season or at change of season?	☐	☐
3. Is it accompanied by bouts of sneezing as well?	☐	☐
4. Do you cough more at night than during the day time?	☐	☐
5. Did you have ezcema in your childhood?	☐	☐

6. Is there a history of bouts of sneezing, eczema or coughing in the family, that is, parents and siblings?

☐   ☐

If the answer to even two of the above questions is in the affirmative, the cough is allergic in nature.

Is your child allergic to a food ?

Yes   No

1. Does the child get a rash around the lips and inside the mouth after taking a particular food?

☐   ☐

2. Does the child have a tendency to throw up a particular food each time it is eaten?

☐   ☐

3. Does the child get abdominal colic?

☐   ☐

4. Is the child losing weight because of inability to retain a particular essential food, for example, milk?

☐   ☐

5. Has the child a reddish oozing rash on the face?

☐   ☐

Interpretation

If your answers are mostly 'Yes', the chances of allergy to an article of food are more.

Seasonal Sneezing or Hay Fever

Bouts of sneezing occurring in a particular season, in medical terminology, is called seasonal allergic rhinitis and in layman's language it is called hay fever. It is the commonest form of allergy. Hay fever does not have any connection with hay. It is the seasonal occurrence of sneezing, a running and congested nose and itching in the eyes and nose. These symptoms occur in a person in a particular season every year, while he feels perfectly normal during the other parts of the year. It may occur in children and in older people, but, it is most common among young people. Males and females are equally effected by it. The symptoms may be mild or very severe and distressing.

Hay fever occurs in those persons who have inherited an allergic tendency. As the pollens to which they are allergic appear in the air in a particular season of the year, the symptoms of the disease occur seasonally.

Symptoms
The onset of sneezing may be gradual or quite sudden, depending on the degree of exposure to the particular

pollens to which the patient is allergic. When the onset is gradual, the attack is usually preceded by a mild sensation of itching and burning of the eyes or mild irritation in the nose or itching of the palate inside the mouth. Attacks of sneezing usually start in the early hours of the morning when there is a sudden increase in the concentration of pollens in the air. Marked nasal congestion and profuse running of the nose and eyes follow the sneezing paroxysms.

As the attack progresses, the nasal mucous membrane becomes highly sensitive and responds with sneezing to small stimuli which were previously innocuous, such as the slightest draft, strong odours, or minute amounts of dust.

Many patients, suffering from hay fever also complain of various constitutional symptoms, such as lassitude, loss of appetite, drowsiness, etc. Some of these symptoms may be due to the self-administration of antihistamine drugs.

Asthma accompaniment

In case of certain people, symptoms of bronchial asthma also appear. They may start at the onset of the disease, or appear later. In certain cases, along with the symptoms of hay fever, there is only a cough and no bronchial spasm. Symptoms of cough and asthma may continue even when attacks of sneezing cease.

Diagnosis of the condition is not difficult and is revealed by the case history.

In the treatment of such cases, it is important to find out the pollen or pollens to which the patient is allergic. This is done by means of skin tests with the extracts of the pollens. Scratch or intracutaneous tests, giving positive reactions for the pollens, coupled with a confirmation of the same through consolidation of the pollen calendar, confirms the causative pollens.

Treatment
Hyposensitisation with the incriminated pollens yields excellent results for this condition.

Role of antihistamines
Symptomatic treatment with antihistamine tablets is very helpful; one has to try one or more kinds of antihistamines to find out which one suits a person particularly well.

Antihistamines have proved most useful in cases of hay fever. Given at the beginning of the attack, they are most effective; they lessen itching, sneezing and running of the nose. Long-acting antihistamines can also be tried in these cases.

Antihistamines come in different forms – tablets, capsules, injections, such as Avil, Phenergan and as mixtures alone or in combination with other drugs such as Actifed and Sudafet.

However, antihistamines are no substitute for a proper detection of the allergens and subsequent hyposensitisation.

Antihistamines should be given only when needed, and not frequently.

In order to prevent the sneezing attacks of hay fever, the following precautions are helpful:

1. Avoid needless outdoor activities during the hay fever seasons.
2. Avoid gardening or farming.
3. If possible, keep bedroom windows closed.

Allergy to Drugs

There has been an increase in the number of drug allergy cases, essentially because of the increased use of a variety of drugs.

All drugs produce some reaction in the body. However, some reactions which are produced are purely allergic in nature. Such unexpected reactions may be due to any of the following causes:

1. Overdosage.
2. Drug interactions, for example, a prescription containing a tranquilliser and an antihistamine may cause excessive drowsiness.
3. Indiscretionary, as for example, an asthmatic may get palpitation of the heart even if he takes just 1/4 gm of ephedrine.
4. Side effects are observed in the form of drowsiness after taking antihistamines.
5. Secondary effects, such as hesitance in passing urine, or even retention of urine on taking ephedrine, that occurs in older people due to an already enlarged prostate.

6. Allergic reactions such as reactions that occur after administration of a drug. In such a case, it is necessary to know its true nature.

Symptoms of an allergic reaction

The first time administration of a drug may cause no adverse reaction initially, but after a few days or weeks there may occur a reaction. Such reactions may occur due to (a) administration, (b) external application, or (c) a person sensitised by external contact may suffer a reaction by later ingestion of the sensitising substance or a related chemical.

Skin lesions

The most common drug reaction is urticaria; others are fever, skin rashes, jaundice and hepatitis. The most severe reaction is of anayphylaxis. Asthma can be one manifestation of reaction.

Urticaria is caused by allergy to various drugs such as penicillin, streptomycin, aspirin, sulphonamides, barbiturates, insulin, liver extract and others. Skin tests are of little use in the diagnosis of the drug responsible for urticaria, the best course being to stop all medication and note the subsequent effects. Contact dermatitis due to drugs allergy has already been described. It may be produced by sulphonamides, antibiotics, local anaesthetics, antihistamines drugs, and many other drugs that are applied on the skin.

Fever

Drug fever is a common complication of treatment with sulphonamides, thiouracil, para-aminosalicylic acid (PAS), arsenicals, and anticonvulsants. The onset typically occurs a week or more after the first use of the drug. The fever may reach to 40^0C and may be continuous or intermittent. When the offending drug is discontinued, the fever subsides as soon as it has been eliminated from the body, usually in a few days.

Blood destruction

Destruction of the blood cells may occur as a result of allergic drug reaction. This may result from the use of aminopyrine, arsenicals, thiouracil, sulphonamides, old and anticonvulsive drugs. Except for old and arsenic, these drugs are rather quickly eliminated from the body and the tendency is to recover within a week of the drug being discontinued.

Allergy to aspirin

The commonly used and innocuous looking aspirin is one of the regular offenders as far as allergic drug reactions are concerned. While most people who take the usual dose of aspirin suffer no immediate ill effects, there are some who are allergic to it and they suffer from a variety of adverse reactions. Skin rashes or urticaria over the whole body or over the eyelid, lips and face are known to occur after taking aspirin. Swelling of the tongue, throat and larynx is sometimes so severe that it leads to suffocation.

Much more serious, however, is the onset of asthma in susceptible persons, after repeated doses of aspirin. Upto 20 percent of severely ill, adult asthma patients have been found to have pairing allergy. Some of these patients are unaware of this until an asthma attack is experimentally provoked in them by giving them test doses of aspirin. Some of the characteristic features of asthma due to aspirin allergy are that persons with aspirin allergy may develop asthma upto three hours after taking the drug. Because of this latent period, many patients fail to connect the taking of aspirin with the subsequent attack. Even after the patient stops taking aspirin, the asthma attacks usually continue. This occurs more frequently in adults than in children. Many patients have nasal polyps. Several asthma patients allergic to aspirin, show positive skin reactions to other allergens as well, such as, pollens and dusts.

Skin tests with aspirin are generally negative; it is only the case history or the experimental trial that helps in the diagnosis of allergy to aspirin.

These patients must be warned of the presence of aspirin in many of the pain-killing and fever relieving tablets and mixtures.

Allergy to vaccines

Various vaccines cause allergic reactions in sensitive people. They also cause some non-allergic reactions and it is essential that a proper differentiation be made between them. Non-allergic reactions include local inflammatory reactions and systemic reactions such as fever, malaise, nausea and vomiting. Allergic reactions may occur in the skin, or the respiratory system, or the nervous system, or the reactions may be anaphylactic in nature. The whooping cough vaccine or the triple vaccine can occasionally cause purpuric rash, fever or shock. Tetanus toxoid has been known to cause urticaria, joint pains or even anaphylactic reactions in patients sensitive to eggs. Antirabic vaccine, in which the virus has been grown on neurological tissue, is known to cause neurological reactions in some individuals. Urticarial rash and increasingly severe local reactions at the injected sites provides indications of impending reaction.

The patient allergic to aspirin, which chemically is acetyl-salicylic acid, is also sensitive to foods which naturally contain salicylates. These are apricots, berries, currants, grapes, peaches, plums, tomatoes and cucumbers. These foods should be avoided by those who are allergic to aspirin.

Diagnosis

The single and most important step is the correct diagnosis of a drug reaction. Some drugs take longer to be eliminated from the body, hence the symptoms of a drug's reaction may continue for a few days after its cessation. Skin tests with drugs are not a reliable guide, and sometimes prove dangerous as well.

Precautions

Symptoms such as fever, general malaise, restlessness or drowsiness, nausea, headache, transient numbness, generalised rashes, oedema, or unusual respiratory symptoms, especially coughing or wheezing are warning symptoms.

Vaccines made of egg, or serum injections made from non-human resources, for example horses, must be given with care, and should be avoided where allergic reactions to them have been noted before. If tetanus toxoid immunisation has been given within five years, do not give ATS, but give a booster dose of 0.5 ml of tetanus toxoid.

The amount and the duration of drug dosage are important. Repeated intermittent administration is more hazardous than continuous administration. The route of administration often effects the sensitising index of the drug. The oral method is least likely to cause sensitisation, the injection more likely, and an application to the skin or mucous membranes is the most likely to cause sensitisation.

Individuals with a family or personal history of allergy, show a greater tendency to develop drug allergies than non-allergic persons; this is particularly true of the immediate reaction. Children are less allergic to drugs than adults. Drugs-sensitised individuals are much more likely to acquire new allergies than those without previous sensitisation.

It is always safe to skin test the patient before giving an injection of an antibiotic, a vaccine or a toxoid. Inject 0.01 ml to 0.02 ml of 1:100 dilution of the drug intradermally into the forearm with a tuberculin syringe (making a small, just visible weal). This can be read in fifteen minutes. Positive reaction consists of swelling (weal), redness and itching. A control test with the same amount of saline solution on a corresponding area of the other arm, at the same time, is also done.

Remember that a negative skin test is not a surety against the occurrence of an allergic drug reaction. If it is positive, the drug is certainly not to be administered.

While giving an injection, avoid the possibility of intravenous inoculation by drawing back on the syringe piston prior to injection. Avoid deposition of vaccine in or near any large nerve trunk.

Treatment

Since most of the manifestations of drug allergy tend to subside as the causative agent is excreted, the most important point of treatment is prompt discontinuation of the medication. For symptomatic treatment of drug allergies, cortisone and allied drugs are the most effective.

Desensitisation is only occasionally helpful. Antihistamine given along with a penicillin injection is a dangerous procedure; antihistamine decreases or prevails upon minor allergic reactions but cannot help severe anaphylactic reactions.

Anaphylactic reaction

A case of anaphylactien shock within seconds or minutes after injection is treated with

1. A tourniquet above the site of injection.
2. Adrenaline 0.5 ml to 1 ml intramuscularly or intravenously, repeated as needed.
3. Antihistamines, but not instead of adrenaline.
4. Artificial respiration and oxygen, if needed.

Penicillin

Allergic reactions to penicillin are very common. They range from urticaria to anaphylaxis; the latter can cause death within minutes.

An anaphylactic reaction to penicillin, generally speaking, begins within seconds or a few minutes after taking it. The following sequence is typical – there is a peculiar taste in the mouth or a sensation in the tongue, and a strange tingling in the extremities. Seconds later, there is severe constriction of the chest, and a choking sensation or dyspnoea develops with increasing rapidity and cyanosis – bluish discolouration of the skin resulting from an increased amount of unoriginated haemoglobin in blood – occurs simultaneously with symptoms of collapse. The whole reaction is sudden and terrifying. Only an alertness to the possible danger and instantaneous availability of the necessary injections and apparatus can save the life of the patient.

Types of reactions

Anaphylactic reaction to penicillin is the most dangerous and the most dramatic; there are others which are less dramatic but more common. These may be categorised as follows:

Delayed reaction

This reaction is the most common one and it is thus called because of its incubation period, usually of 7 to 11 days; the minimum may be five days and the maximum perhaps about eight weeks. It is the response to initial sensitisation and not to the previous exposure to penicillin. Ulticaria is by far the most common symptom; others are joint pains, malaise and fever.

Accelerated and immediate reactions

These reactions are much less frequent and occur only in patients who have been sensitised by previous exposure to penicillin. The accelerated reactions appear in a few hours or in two to three days, and the immediate type occurs within seconds or minutes or within two hours. Clinically, these vary from the mild to the, more often, severe. There may be urticaria, breathlessness and anaphylaxis.

Hyperallergic reactions

These are rare and include more intense and accelerated reactions with bullous eruptions – a thin walled air-filled space within the lung, arising congenitally or in emphysema.

Contact dermatitis

This follows the topical application of penicillin in the ointment form, but can manifest itself with other forms of application as well. The eruption may be acute, or chronic.

Indirect reactions

Patients sensitive to penicillin are known to get reactions from it even from indirect sources. If a cow or a buffalo has been given a penicillin injection, even drinking its milk, by a patient sensitive to penicillin, is known to cause reactions. Some of the chronic reactions, such as urticaria may be perpetuated by penicillin through such indirect and often undetected sources.

Anaphylactic reaction to penicillin can occur not only after penicillin given by injection but also when it is administered orally in the form of a tablet, or instilled into the eye, ears or nose, or when applied on the skin as an ointment.

Those with a significant occurrence of asthma in their families, and a similar personal history of either asthma or hay fever, usually have a higher incidence of penicillin reaction. Children show a lesser incidence of penicillin allergy than adults.

The commonest reaction to penicillin is appearance of rash all over the body.

Skin test with penicillin

A positive skin test, observed at 15 minutes and most safely elicited by the scratch method, is a definite warning signal of potential anaphylaxis. When the case history suggests the possibility of anaphylaxis, the test is most safely carried out with graded dilutions beginning with 100 units per ml. and increasing to 50,000 units per ml. If the scratch test is negative, then intracutaneous tests may be carried out with dilutions of penicillin varying from 1000 to 50,000 units per ml., employing 0.2 ml., as is done in star allergy testing, to produce a just visible test weal.

The positive delayed skin test reaction, read like a tuberculin test (to know whether a person is infected with TB germs) after 24 to 48 hours, for redness and swelling in the skin occurs in those who have had a previous reaction to penicillin. This reaction is some times associated with urticaria or minute eruptions.

A careful note should be made of the fact that a negative skin test is no guarantee against adverse reactions to penicillin.

Prevention

Penicillin should not be used unless absolutely necessary. Before prescribing or injecting penicillin, a careful history should be taken as to (a) the frequency of previous penicillin treatments as it is the repeated exposure to this antibiotic that is more likely to result in shock, (b) any evidence of a previous allergic reaction to the antibiotic, (c) personal history of allergy and especially of bronchial asthma, and (d) skin test by scratch method must be done.

Paradoxically, however, most patients who get anaphylactic shock have no past history of previous penicillin allergy.

An injection is best given in the outer arm rather than in the buttock or deltoid so that, if need be, a tourniquet can be applied proximally to delay absorption.

Treatment

In anaphylaxis, adrenaline 0.5 to 1.0 ml. is administered subcutaneously. It works as the most effective antidote; in extreme urgency. A tourniquet should, if possible, be applied proximal to the injection site to delay absorption. The patient is placed in a recumbent position and if necessary, oxygen may be given with a bronchodilator through intermittent positive pressure breathing. Injection of antihistamine and intravenous cortisone can be helpful.

Desensitisation with penicillin is too hazardous in patients with a history of an immediate or anaphylactic reaction.

Those who are allergic to penicillin or its derivatives may also be allergic to related drugs like ampicillin and amoxycillin.

Emergency Kit

Adrenaline	1 ml. ampoules of 1:1000-five 30 ml. Vial of 1 : 1000.
Aminophylline	Ampoules of aminophylline of 250 mg. each.
Deriphylline	1 ml. ampoules for 1/m injection-5.

Antihistamines	One 10 ml. vial of injectable (50 mg / ml).
	Avil tabs 25 mg. each -10 tabs.
Steroids	Decadron 2 ml. vial. -5 vials.
	Betnalan tabs -50 tabs.
	Prednisolone tabs -50
Syringes	Tuberculin syringes -2
	2 ml all - glass syringes -2 with needles.
Tourniquet	